Special Dedication to Our Friends

Saffron

Willoughby

Jorie

Zack

Micah

Logan

Caroline

Healthy Hellos: Fun & Healthy Greetings - No Handshakes Needed!
© 2025
by Morrison Parfet, Cortland Parfet, and Bo Parfet

Illustrations by Kai Sersoseh
Character Design & Art Direction by Bo Parfet

Paperback ISBN: 979-8-9874372-3-0
Ebook ISBN: 979-8-9874372-4-7

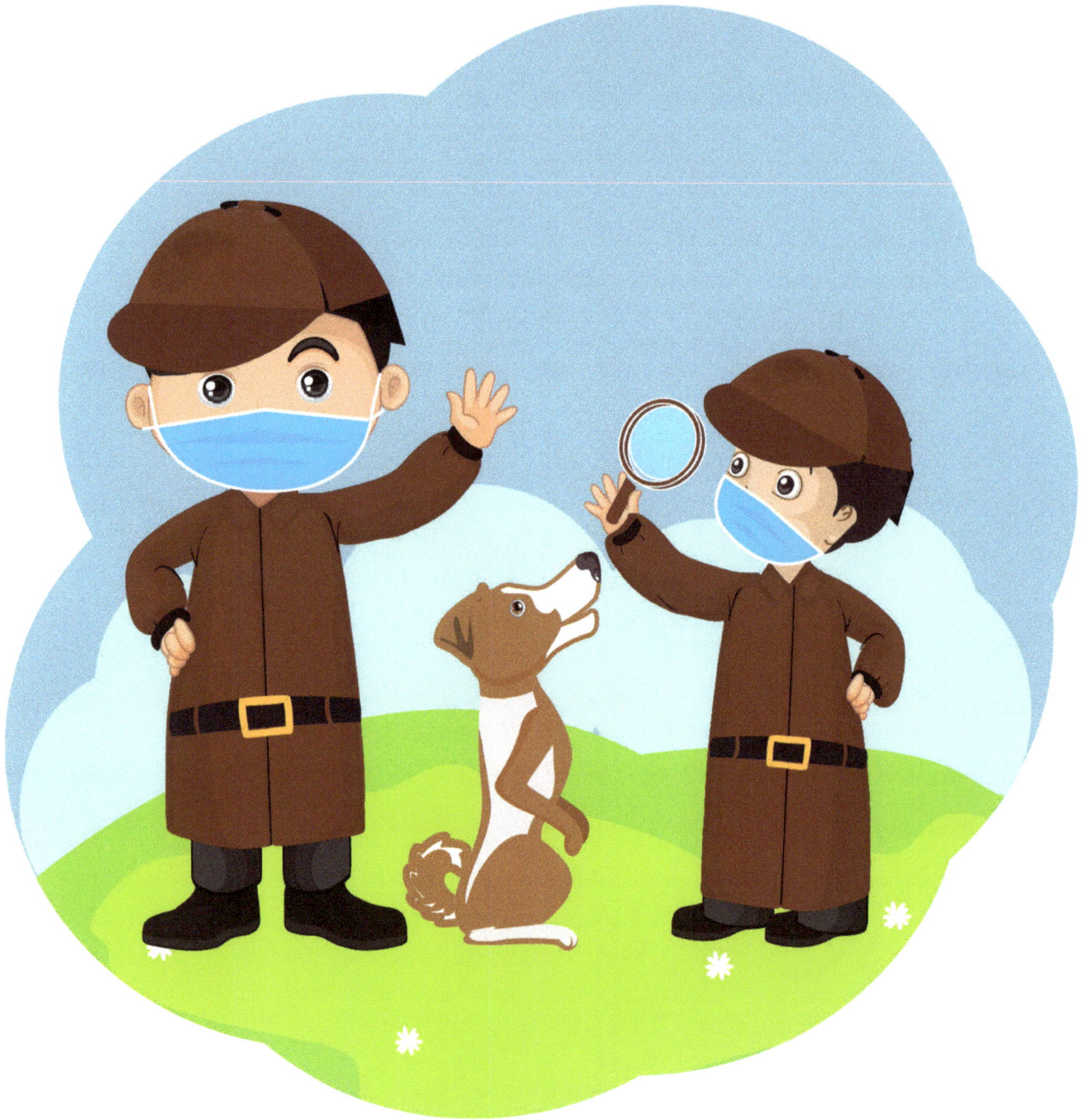

Momo P.I., Miss Poodle Pants & Coco

Hi! I'm Mo and with me, as always, is my brother Cortland. I love to learn about the world and use what I learn to help people who are in tricky situations. That's why my Grandma Zizi calls me Mo P.I. The P.I. stands for private investigator. Investigating life all around me is what I love to do.

Normally, I'd shake your hand, but, as you probably know, life has been pretty different since the year 2020. A dangerous virus known as COVID-19 spread to people all around the world. While COVID-19 created a lot of havoc in our lives, it has also raised our awareness of how viruses are spread.

To keep people safe, we wore masks in public, did not greet one another with handshakes, and used lots of hand sanitizer. These are good things to practice all the time because viruses, even colds, are easily spread to others through the moisture on our hands and in our mouths and noses. When we sneeze, cough, or even talk to one another, little droplets of moisture escape.

And, if we touch our mouths or noses, moisture (aka germs) is transferred to our hands. Germs can even enter through our eyes if we rub them after touching a person — or even a doorknob or shopping cart. That's why we don't shake hands and why we do use hand sanitizer.

Today, I will focus on handshakes because of something my brother, Cortland, recently asked me. He said, "Mo, if people can't shake hands, what can we do to greet other people?"

That's a great question! As someone who likes to observe the world, I've done some research on how people from around the world say "hello." Be sure to pay attention because I'll be asking you if the greeting is safe — or not.

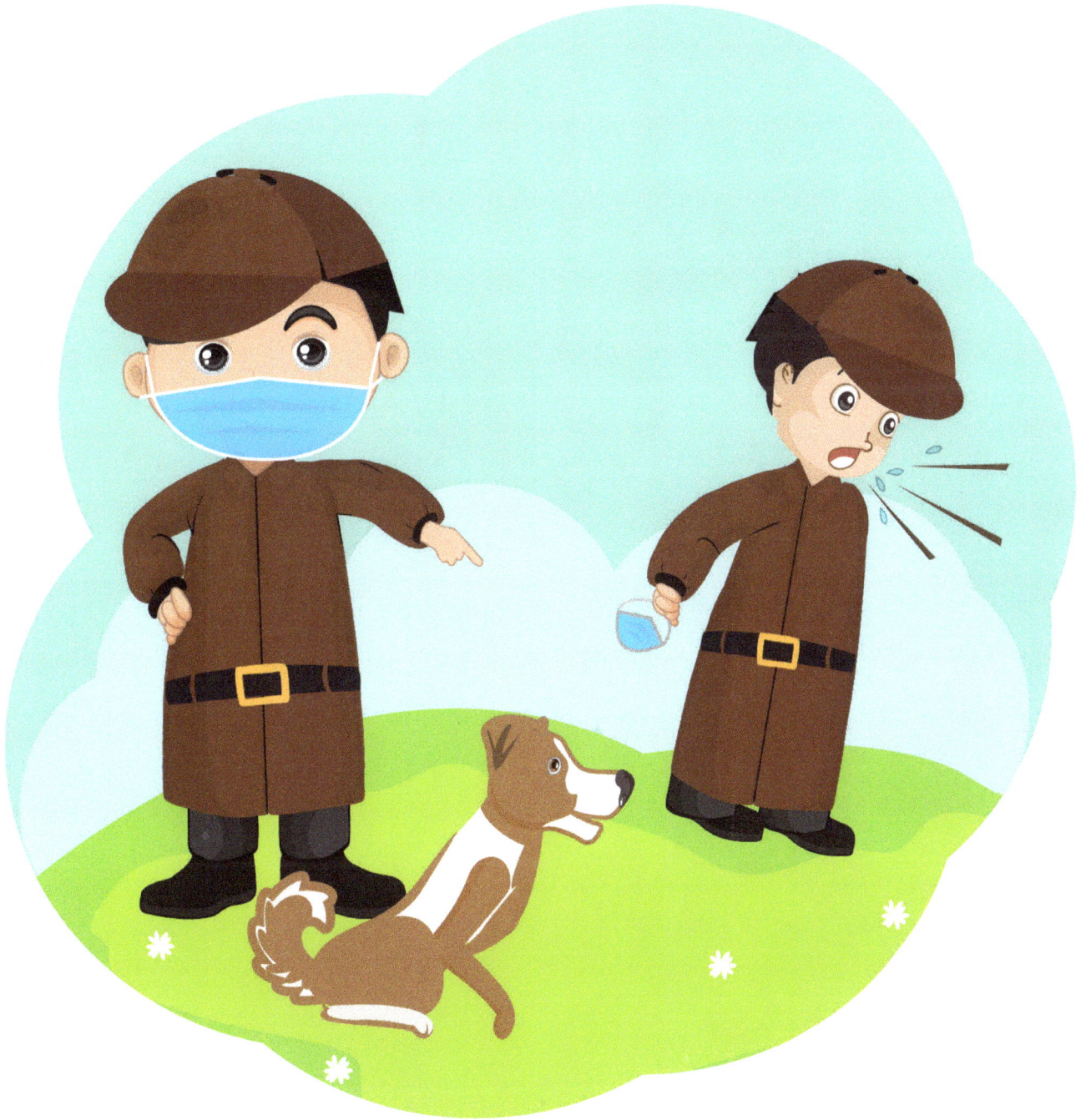

The mask can cover up the sneeze.

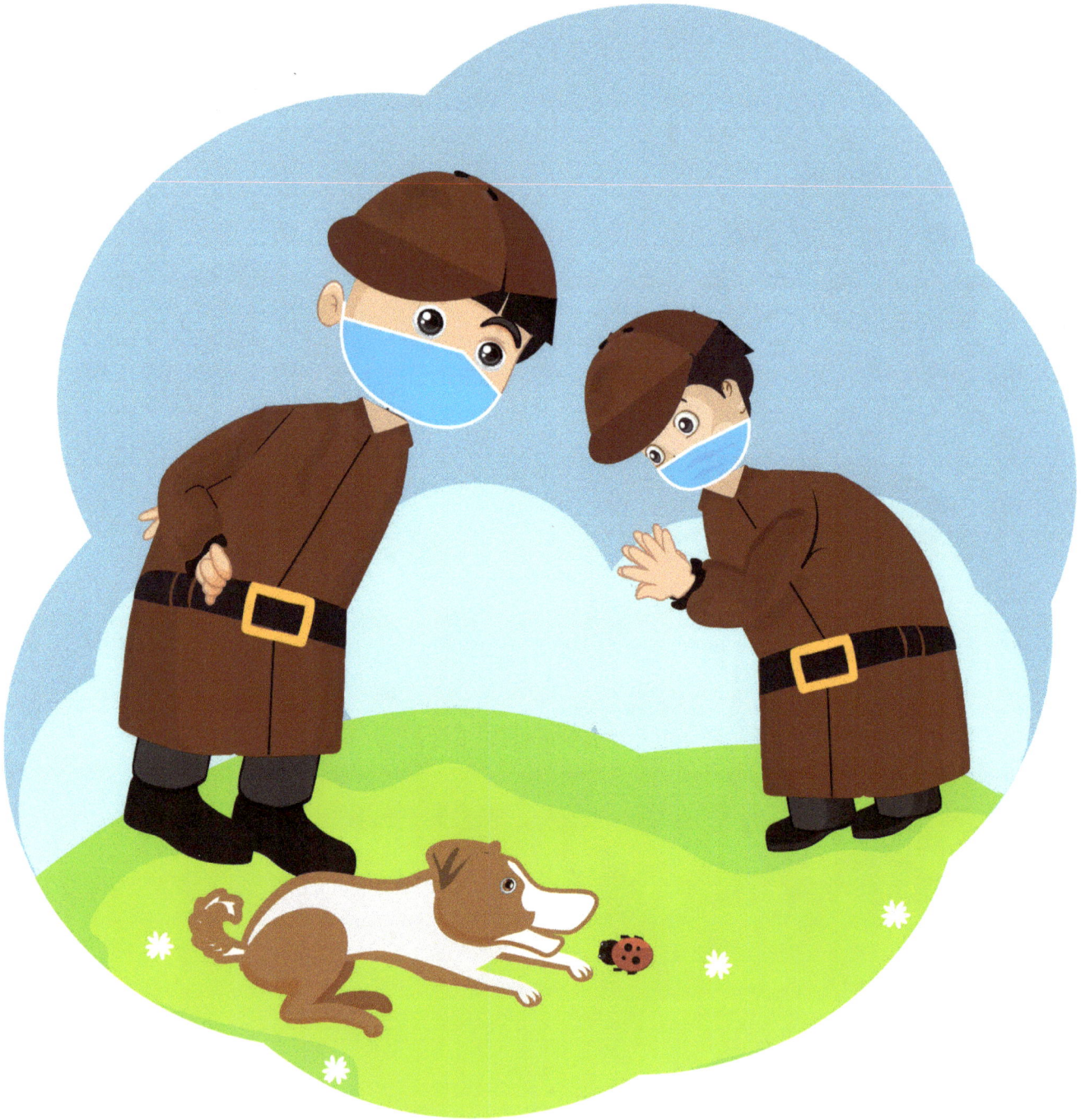

Even though they're not touching, Mo P.I. and Cortland are still wearing masks for safety.

In some cultures, like Japan, people greet each other by bowing. They bend at the waist, with their hands by their sides, and lower their upper body toward the person in front of them. In Thailand, people press their hands together in front of their hearts. Both are signs of kindness or respect.

So, what do you think? Would this be a Healthy Hello?

If you said, "Yes," you'd be right, as long as the people don't get too close. Bowing involves no touching and can be done from a distance. Give it a try right now!

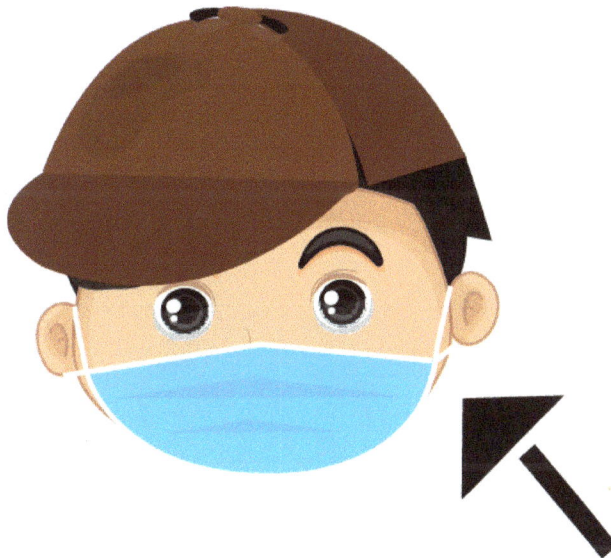

Make sure your mask is pulled up above your nose.

Let's try another. Sometimes, you'll see people tap their knuckles against someone else's knuckles. This is a fist bump. It's a common greeting between people who know each other well in the United States. We often congratulate someone on a job well done, like running a race or winning a game, with a fist bump. The origin of the fist bump is unclear. Some say it started when boxers used to bump their gloves against each other before a boxing match.
Is this a germ-free way of saying hello?

What do you think?

Fist-bumping isn't safe. Even though there is less moisture on your knuckles than in the palm of your hand, germs can still be spread when someone's skin touches someone else's skin. The person you're fist-bumping might have just coughed into their hand, and you wouldn't know! Also, you must get close to a person to do a fist bump.

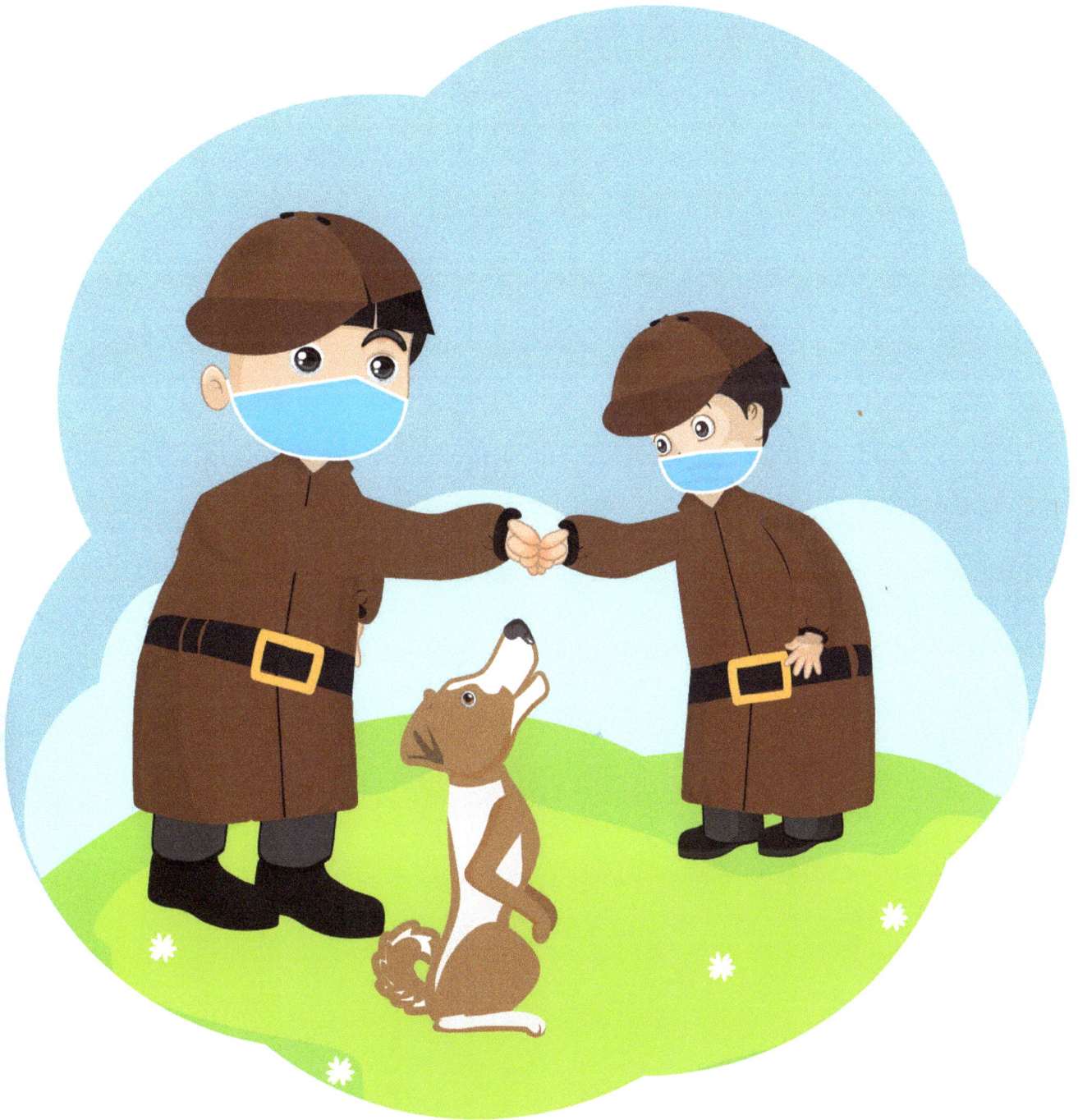

Miss Poodle Pants wants a closer look as the boys touch knuckles.

Did you know that in some cultures, people greet each other by rubbing noses? No one is sure how this tradition started, but it's been around for hundreds of years. Saudi Arabia is one country where you might see people rub noses when they greet. The Indigenous people of Alaska, the Inuits, have a name for rubbing noses — kinuk. The Māori of New Zealand press their noses together, and it's referred to as hongi.

This greeting may have been around for a long time, but is it safe now?

That's a definite "no."

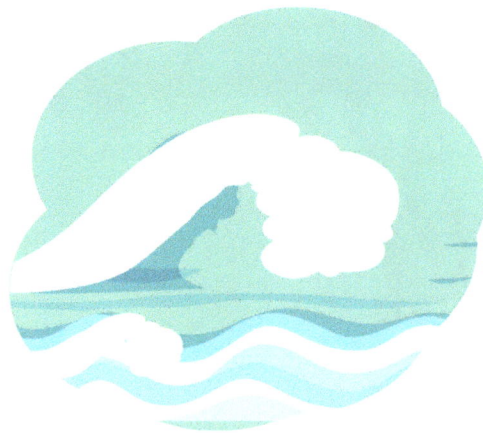

Here is a good joke you can tell your friends:
- How does the ocean say hello?
- It waves!

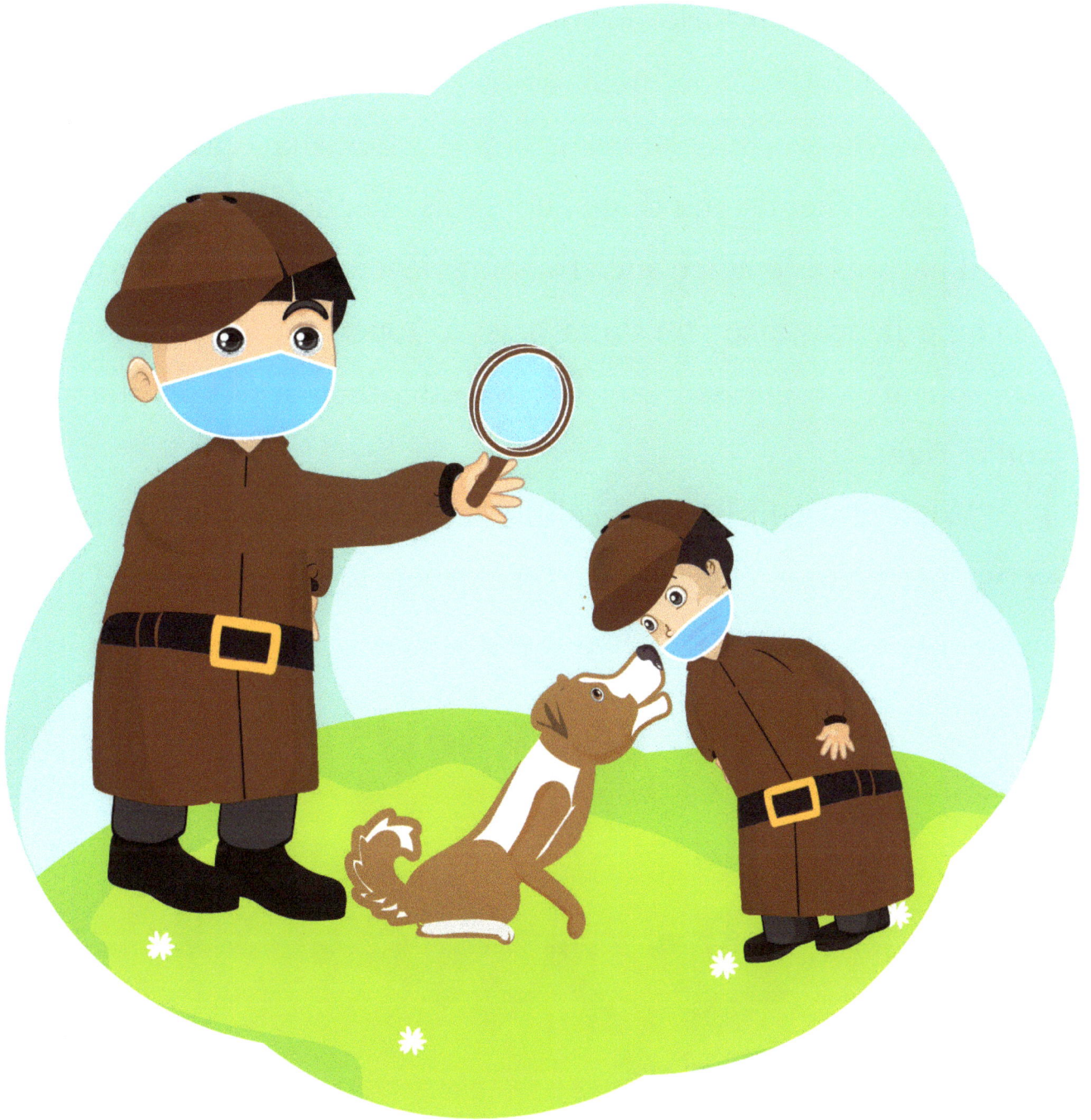

Miss Poodle Pants has a wet nose!

The next one is tricky, so you'll want to give this some thought. Since the COVID-19 outbreak, some people have begun greeting each other by touching shoes or doing a foot shake instead of a handshake. What do you think about this one? Is it safe?

That was a tougher one. Touching feet is certainly safer than touching hands since you don't have to touch the other person's skin, but if you guessed that it's not safe, then it's "safe" to say you're right.

While it might be the healthier option, you still need to get very close to another person to touch their foot with yours. That would put you within the coughing or sneezing range.

DID YOU KNOW?

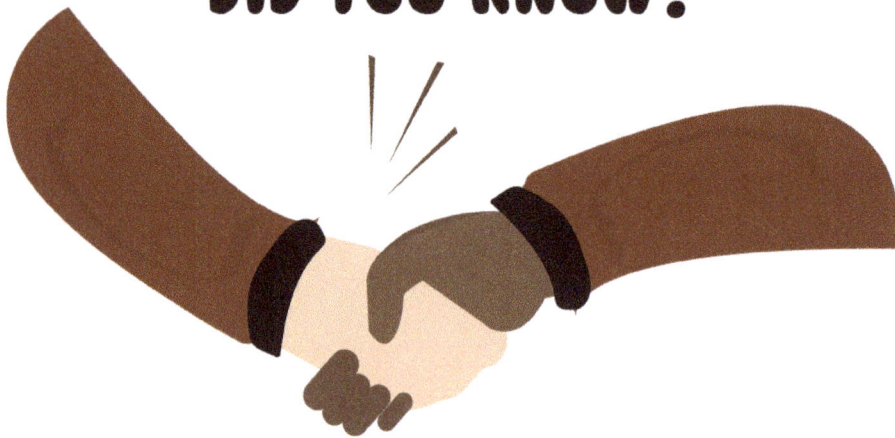

An average person will shake hands 1,500 times in their lifetime.

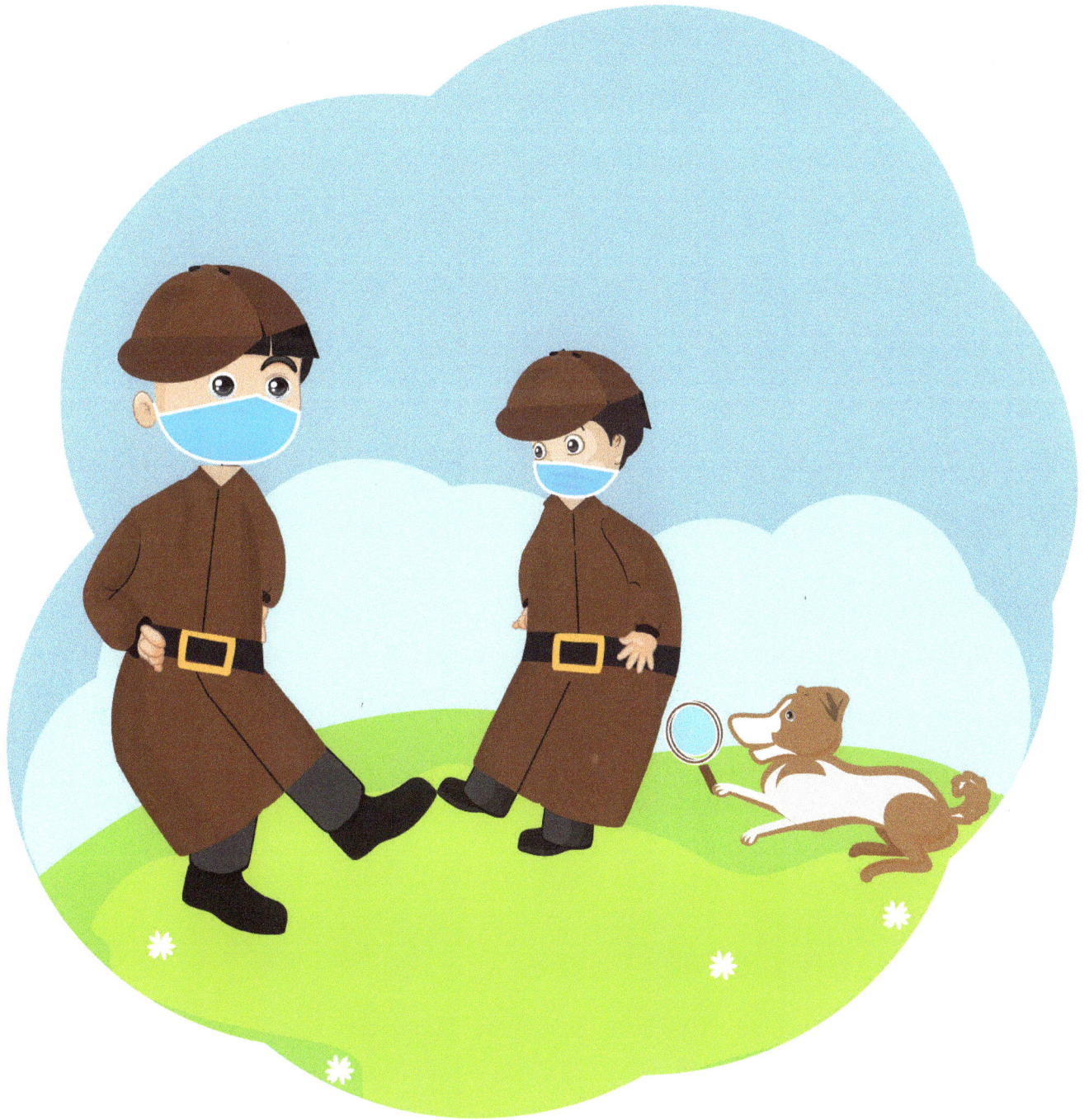

The boys are touching shoes, but Miss Poodle Pants thinks they are dancing.

Let's try another. What about placing your hand over your heart and giving a small nod? Does this seem like a safe way to greet another person?

That one is definitely safe. You don't have to touch another person, and you can do it from a distance. People place their hands on their hearts to show that they are honest and sincere. It can also demonstrate that what they are saying comes from their heart, which means it comes from a place of kindness and love.

The head nod is like a small bow. It, too, demonstrates kindness and respect. So, when you greet someone with a nod and place your hand on your heart, you are greeting the other person with love and respect.

Give it a try right now!

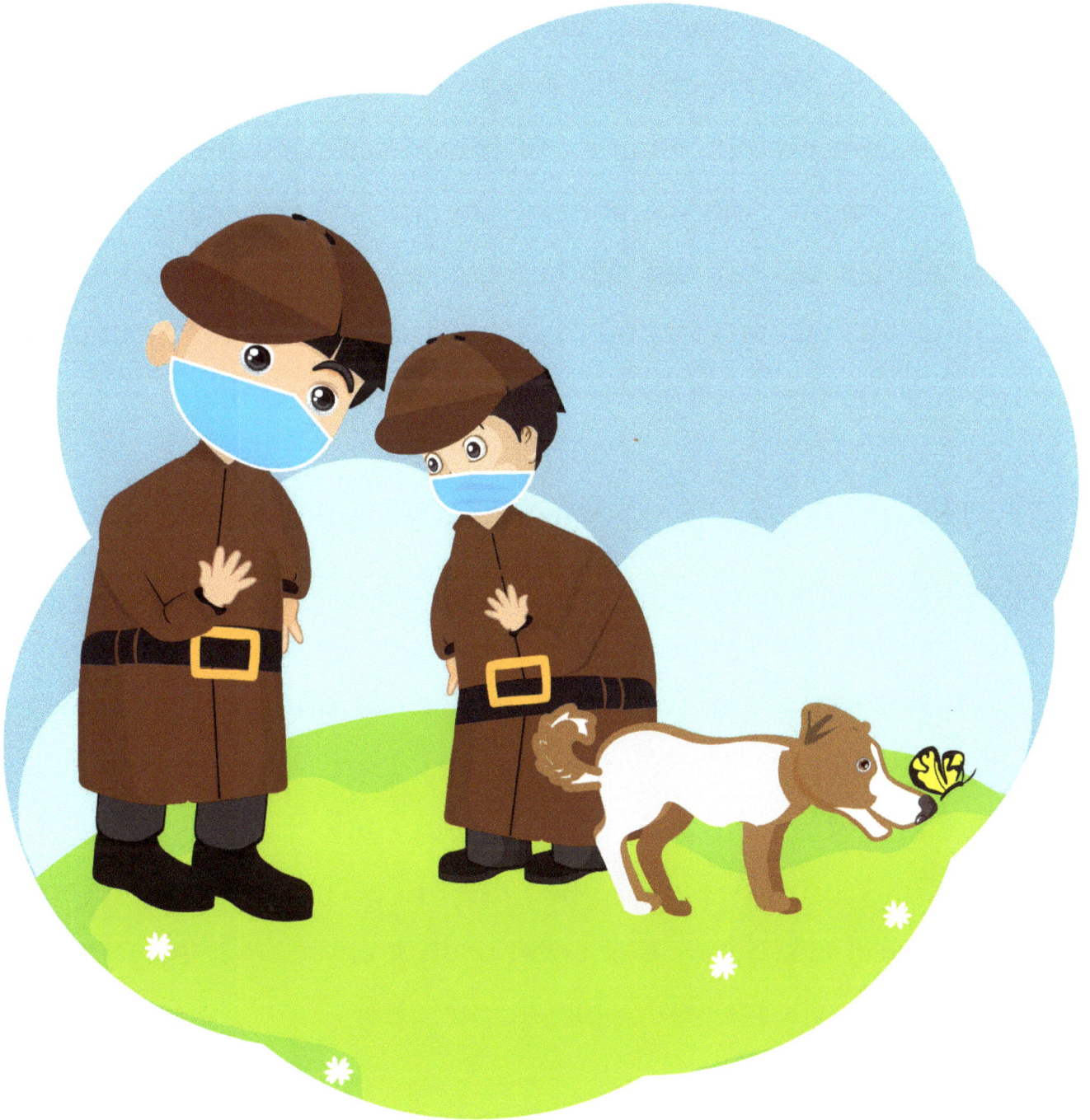

The boys place their hands on their hearts and
wave towards each other.

Here's another greeting that is very common in many cultures: kisses on the cheek. This is seen in many countries around the world. However, the number of kisses varies depending on the country. In many South American countries, the greeting is one kiss on the cheek. In some Middle Eastern and European countries, it's two, first one side and then the other. Then there are those European countries that share three kisses upon meeting.

This greeting is certainly very popular worldwide, but is it safe right now?

If you said, "no," you're right. Viruses can spread quickly through the mouth. If someone is ill, you don't want to kiss them. You could practice this right now on your stuffed animal, though! And here's the tricky part, sometimes the germs are active even before we feel sick! So, we don't ever really know if we're spreading germs. That's why it's best to play it safe!

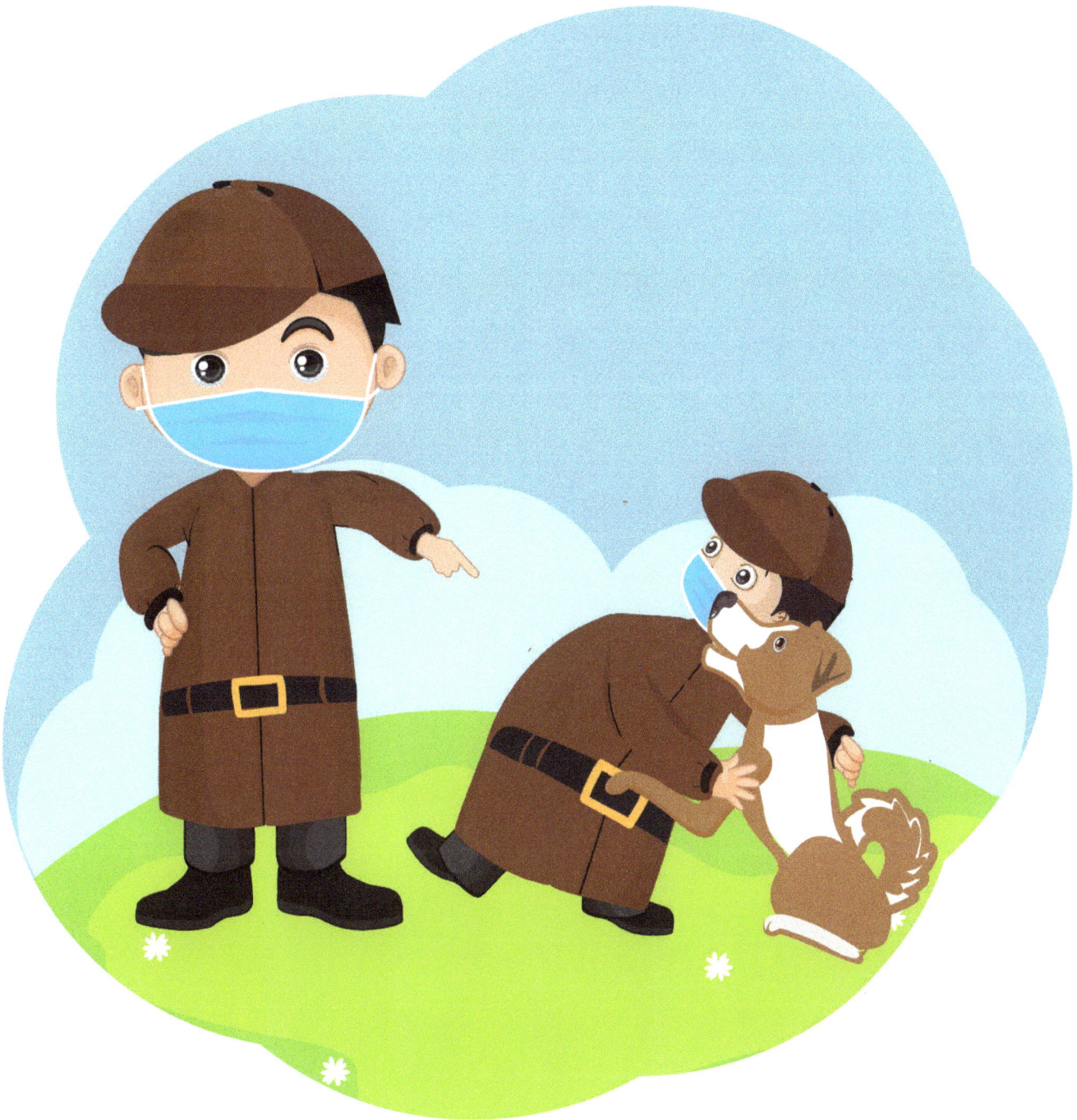

Miss Poodle Pants is giving Cortland a kiss on the cheek.

Finally, what about an air salute, like an air high-five or an air hug? This is where you pretend to high-five or hug someone, but you do it from a distance, so you don't actually touch them.

That was an easy one. And the answer, of course, is yes; it's safe. Since you're not touching the other person, and you are standing at a safe distance. Other air salutes are a thumbs-up and, of course, the good old-fashioned wave.

Give it a try right now!

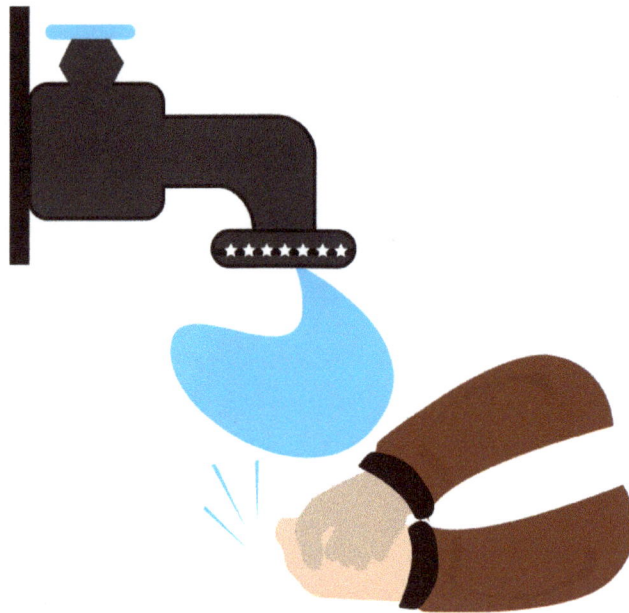

Washing your hands regularly is another way to stay safe.

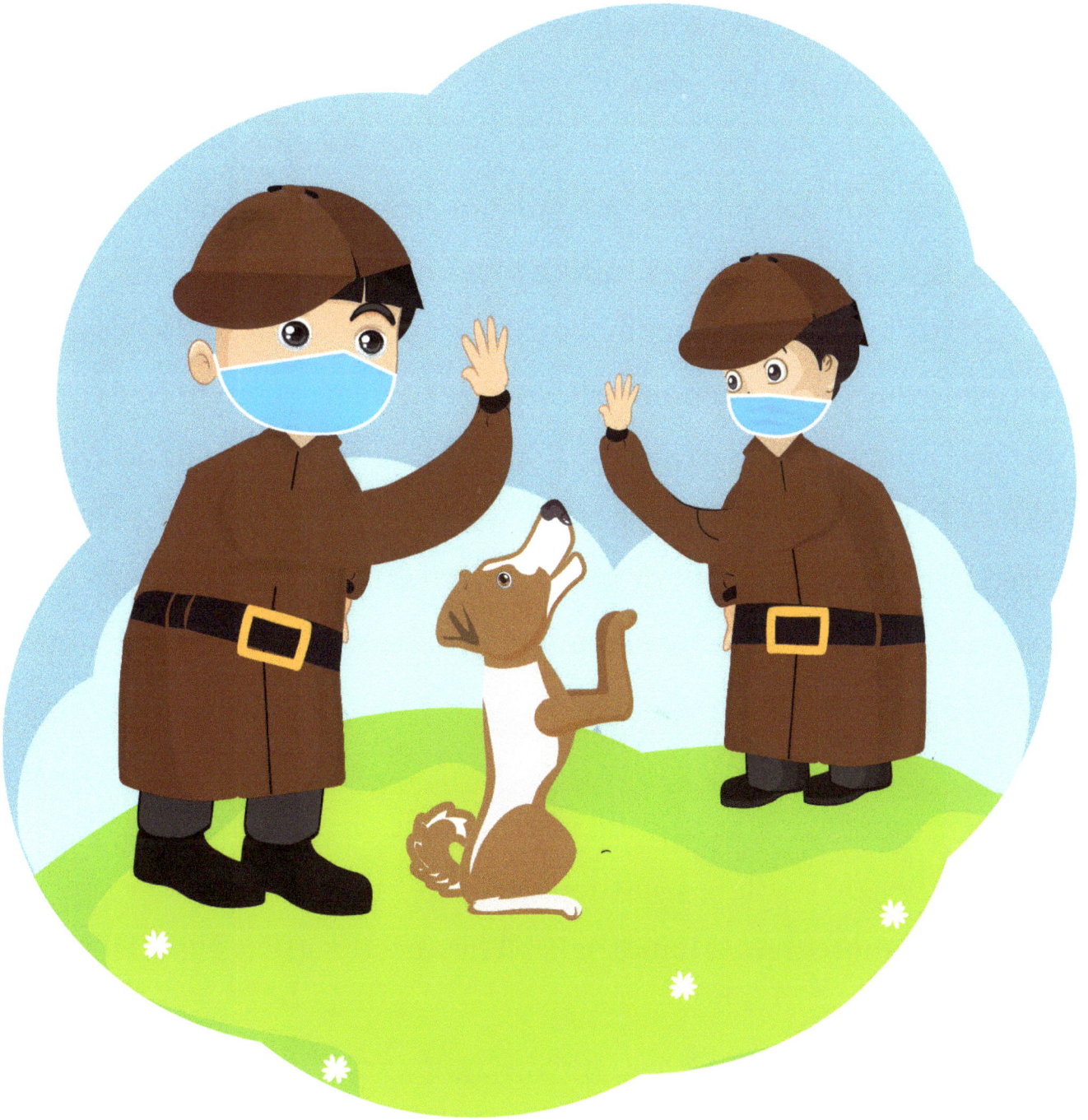

The boys keep distance between their hands for an air high-five.

So, here you have some great, safe ways to greet other people. Great job figuring those out!

Before I go, I wanted to share a great question Cortland asked me. "Why is shaking hands a common greeting?"

The handshake actually goes back more than 2,000 years! People would clasp each other's hands or forearms to check to see if they were carrying weapons. If you shook someone's hand, you showed them you did not have a weapon. So, in a way, people originally shook hands to prove they were safe! How funny is that? Now, at times, we avoid shaking hands to be safe.

How the world has changed!

Fortunately, there are still some people we can get close to — like the person reading you this book right now. For those people, they need more than a handshake. They need a great big HUG!

Bye-bye from Mo P.I. and Cortland!

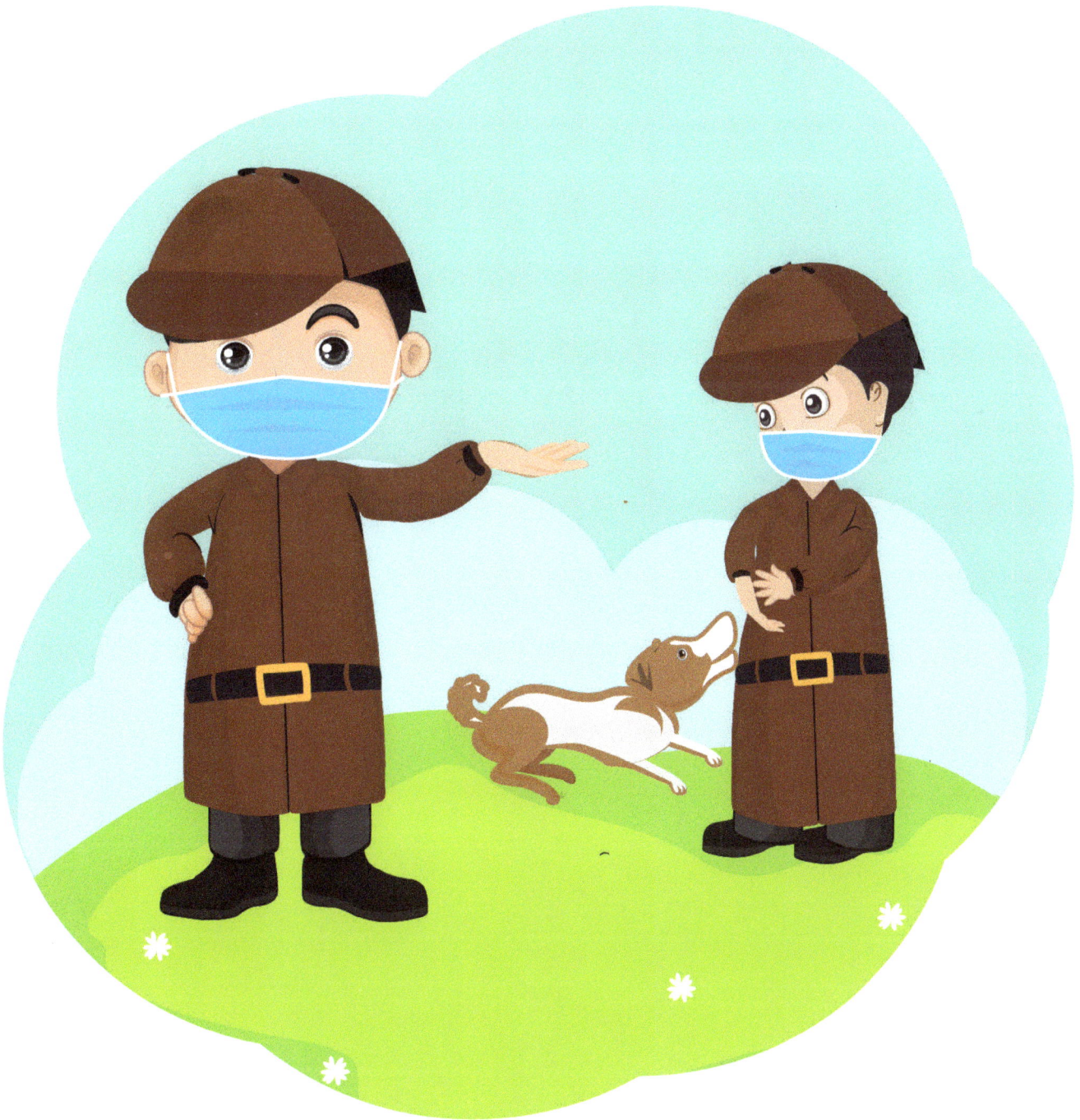

Cortland has nothing up his sleeve!

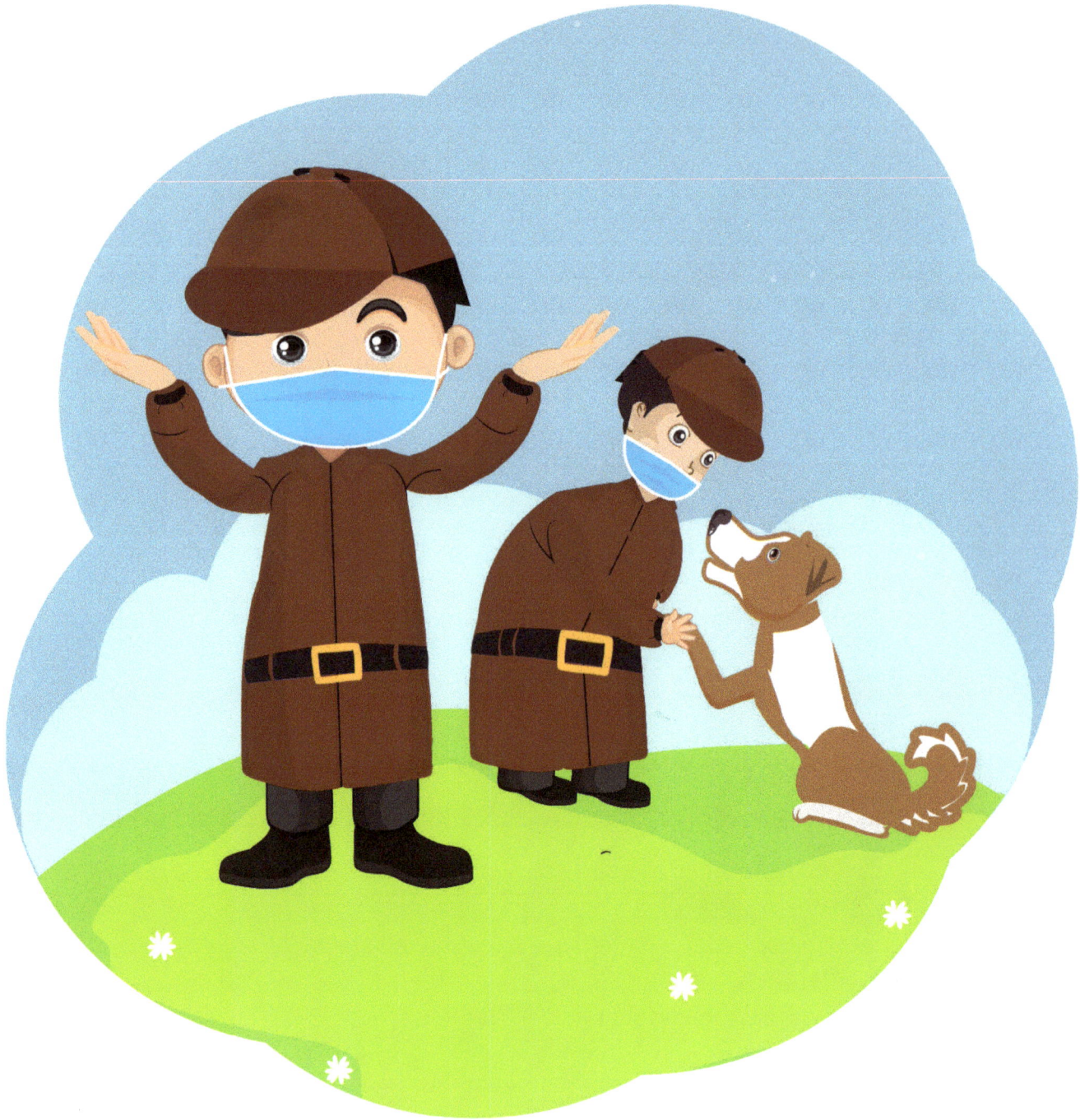

It's okay for Cortland to shake hands with Miss Poodle Pants. Dogs aren't known to have the virus.

ABOUT THE AUTHORS

Morrison "Mo" Parfet is the older brother of Cortland, and they are close friends. Mo enjoys skiing, rock climbing, adventure travel, reading, and much more.

Cortland Parfet is the younger brother of Mo. Cortland loves skiing, biking, rock climbing, adventure travel, and reading Harry Potter books.

Bo Parfet is a proud father to both Mo and Cortland. He enjoys sharing outdoor adventures with his boys. The family lives in Colorado with Mom Meredith.

www.ingramcontent.com/pod-product-compliance
Lightning Source LLC
Chambersburg PA
CBHW041602260326
41914CB00011B/1361